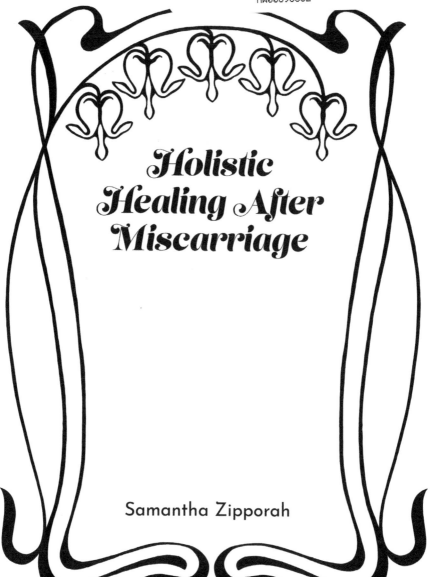

Holistic Healing After Miscarriage

Samantha Zipporah

I

Acknowledgments

I have immense gratitude for the guidance & support I received weaving this content from:

Angela Carter ND
Lara Pacheco Clinical Herbalist seedandthistle.com
Molly Dutton-Kenny CPM mollyduttonkenny.com

Disclaimer

This booklette is meant to be used to facilitate holistic healing following a miscarriage. It is not meant to replace professional or clinical care when needed, desired, or appropriate. Many people experiencing miscarriage may also benefit from clinical care to assess bleeding, infection prevention, & assured completion of miscarriage.

Holistic Healing After Miscarriage 2nd Edition

© 2019 Samantha Zipporah

Table of Contents

Introduction

Miscarriage is a universally common experience that needs
respect, community, support, & dialogue.

- 10–25% of pregnancies end in miscarriage during the first
  20 weeks of a pregnancy.

- Up to 50% of miscarriages occur during the first month of
  pregnancy.

- The primary "cause" of miscarriage is genetic abnormality in
  growth of the embryo.

- Only about 1% of people will have multiple subsequent
  miscarriages.

Too many people experience miscarriage in isolation & without
holistic care. A holistic model of care is one that acknowledges
the interconnectedness of our mind, body, & spirit as an inte-
grated whole. We have compiled the information in this booklette to support individual self-care & as a guide for friends,
family, & community.

Amidst the likelihood of pain & grief, miscarriage presents an
opportunity for profound transformation & reverence for life.
The womb is a spirit door. In regaining balance from pregnancy
loss we have the opportunity to intentionally examine, define, &
manifest our connection with divine creative energy implicit in
our bodies.

Though the compartmentalization of the mind, body, & spirit
is a dangerous & disempowering illusion, I have used these
categories as a convenient way to organize content. Since these
dimensions of self-overlap, many of the suggestions will apply to
more than one category.

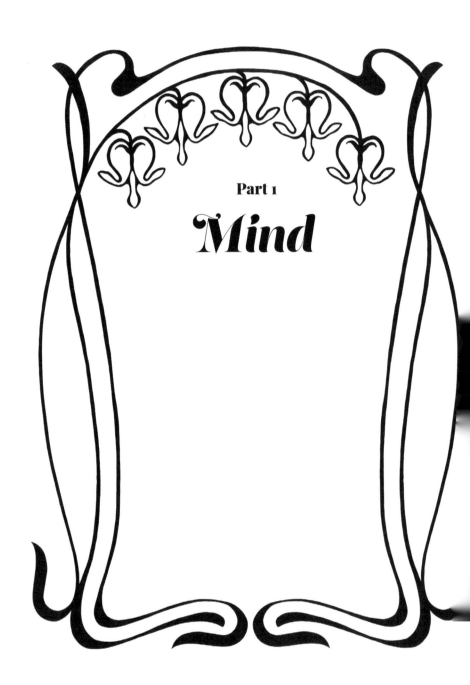

Part 1
Mind

It is totally normal for our minds & emotions to take longer to heal than our bodies after pregnancy loss. Here are some suggestions to help you find peace of mind & balance:

Radical Self Acceptance

Give yourself permission to think or feel your unique personal truth.

There is no right or wrong way to think or feel about your experience.

Claim it, own it, express it, let it out.

"Every emotion that you feel is real. It is truth. It comes directly from the integrity of your spirit. You cannot fake what you feel. You can try to justify or repress your emotions, you can try to lie about what you feel, but what you feel is authentic. There are no good emotions or bad emotions. Even if what you feel is anger or hate, it comes from your integrity. If you feel it, there is always a reason for feeling it."

Don Miguel Ruiz "The Voice of Knowledge"

Many people experiencing miscarriage, & their supporters & community, may feel a wide variety of emotions. For some of us, naming & deeply feeling each emotion allows us to honor it, feel it to its fullest, & let it go when we're ready. Some of these emotions may include:

- Numbness

- Ambivalence

- Grief, Loss, Sadness

- Guilt

- Regret

- Anger

- Shame, Rage

- Confusion

- Betrayal, Abandoned

- Empty, Depleted

- Weary, Exhausted

- Relief

- Peace

- Gratitude

- Connectedness

If you are having trouble processing emotions, consider reading through this list & lingering on the most salient suggestions of emotions you may be feeling. Resting your hand on your heart & your womb, breathe slowly in & out, focusing on feeling one emotion at a time or a beautiful mixture. Take the time you need to feel.

This is by no means an exhaustive list. Each individual is unique & will add or subtract to this list as they see fit, & some feelings are unnamable.

Finding Your Personal Truth

Take note of where your thoughts are coming from. Are they yours? Are you harboring beliefs from your culture or family that you don't really identify with? Are you suffering from projections & causing yourself anguish? If you find yourself having thoughts or feelings that you feel are invasive or not your own, acknowledge them, let them go, & check in with your center to see what is actually true for you.

Get Support

Breaking the pattern of isolation that is prevalent with pregnancy loss is so important. In addition to reaching out to talk with loved ones or others in your community, you may want to seek the support of a professional counselor or therapist. There are a lot of amazing support networks online as well, check out the resource section of this booklette.

Support may also be sought from those traditionally viewed as "birth workers": local midwives, doulas (especially "full spectrum" doulas), & others who support pregnancy experiences. While many of these community members are best known for their work with birth, most also have extensive training, experience, & resources for miscarriage.

Gather Stories

Read the stories of others & know that you are not alone. In addition to the many websites listed in the resource section, I particularly love the stories shared in Christiane Northrup's book *Women's Bodies, Women's Wisdom*.

Forgiveness & Self-Love

Many people experiencing miscarriage will question what more they could have done to support the pregnancy, or wonder why the pregnancy/spirit ended at this time. Common misconceptions perpetuated by public impression may leave us feeling like the miscarriage was our fault.

In reality, most miscarriages are entirely spontaneous & no amount of changed habits, thoughts, lifestyle or other efforts could have prevented the outcome.

Some of the most important efforts toward healing & integration may be in the form of simple self-love & self-acceptance. Accepting that the miscarriage was not your fault, radiate forgiveness, acceptance, love, & understanding inward.

Extend to yourself the great care you would extend to a friend in the same situation.

Homeopathics

Homeopathic remedies are energy medicine & consist of extremely high dilutions of various medicinal elements. Homeopathy is based on the idea that the body can heal itself with subtle support, as well as the principle that you can treat "like with like," meaning that a very small dose of a substance that would create specific symptoms in a healthy person will be healing of those specific symptoms in somebody who is unwell. Homeopathic remedies can be used to address physical as well as emotional symptoms & are best prescribed from an experienced homeopath.

Homeopathic remedies are most commonly available in tiny sweet pills that are placed under the tongue to dissolve, but may also be available as tinctures, creams, & other preparations. The container of tiny sweet pills should be percussed, or shaken against the palm of the hand, before use to "activate" the energetic properties, & should be deposited directly from the container under the tongue, not touched with our fingers.

Sabina
To help expel retained products of conception, especially with excessive, painful bleeding.

Arnica
For shock & injury, a uterus with profuse red bleeding.

Staphysagria
Deep emotional, unforgivable guilt, apologetic, trying to make amends, sexual conflicts.

Caulophyllum
To aid in regulating contractions when contractions are sharp, spasmodic, low in pelvis, & associated with shaking, weakness, or nervous excitement.

Cimicifuga

To aid in regulating contractions through uterine dysfunction alongside negativity, morbid fears, & fragmented thoughts.

Pulsatilla

Easy changeability or emotions influenced easily by others, very cold or very hot in environment, possible restlessness or indigestion, weepy, apologetic, desiring company.

Ammonium Muriaticum

Tearful & grieving, but can't cry. Doesn't want to talk, irritable & angry.

Apis mellifica

Depression & antipathy. Cannot help but cry. Foggy thinking—can't concentrate, mind feels paralyzed. Sudden crying out during sleep.

Aurum Metallicum

Self condemning & feelings of worthlessness. Depression & hopelessness with suicidal ideation. Very sensitive to stimuli. Does not respond well to contradiction.

Causticum

Grief with suppressed emotion. Hypochondria, fearful, restless apprehension, especially at night. Highly sensitive.

Gelsemium Sempervirens

Grief with irritation. Does not want to be spoken to, wants to be left alone. Dullness & confusion. Weeping.

Ignatia Amara

Silent intense anger, sadness, & grief with much sighing. Preference for solitude. Emotional tenderness. Haunting guilt.

Natrum Muriaticum

Preference for grieving & crying alone. Cravings for salt & the ocean. Feels worse with consolation. Irritable & reactive. Deep guilt.

Phosphoricum acidum

Indifference. Not interested in the world or life. Sadness & foreboding about the future. Cannot endure noise or conversation.

Flower Essences

Flower Essences are liquid vibrational medicine made from flowers, spring water, & a tiny bit of alcohol as a preservative, often infused in sunlight. Their process in the body is similar to acupuncture, reiki, & homeopathy. See www.flowersociety.org for more info.

Love Lies Bleeding
Assists with extreme physical & psychic pain. Indicated when person feels as though they have been taken to their absolute limit, Love Lies Bleeding helps with spiritual transformation.

Water Violet
For grief with isolation. Helps to bring deep feelings to the surface & to process them, helps come out of hiding & back into community.

Honeysuckle
For people lost in rumination & memory of lost loved ones. Helps with perspective & presence, ability to move on.

Gentian
Comforting to the heart & hope, to help restore faith that life is overall good.

Olive
Exhaustion, long illness &/or emotional struggle within the household following a death. Restores emotional energy & thus physical energy /stamina.

Hornbeam
When grief drains one's enthusiasm about life, simply not having the energy, interest, or enthusiasm to start the day.

Star of Bethlehem
For trauma followed by shock. A good alternative to rescue remedy in situations without panic.

Mariposa Lily

Helps create access to & peace with the inner Divine Feminine & Mother.

Rescue Remedy

A mix of five flower essences: Impatiens, Star of Bethlehem, Cherry Plum, Rock Rose, & Clematis. To be used in "emergency" emotional situations to help calm nerves & bring peace. Not for extended use.

My absolute favorite tool for healing an anxious or unhappy mind is a simple yet profound shift in perspective:

Transform worrying to wondering
&
concern to curiosity.

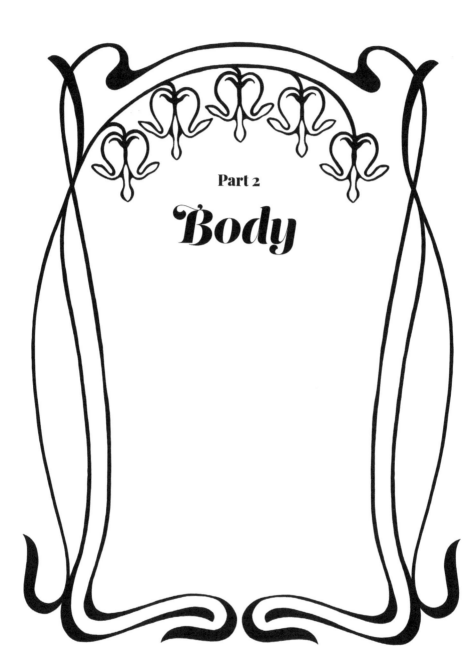

Part 2

Body

I do not give specific dosage recommendations for herbs or remedies, as each individual's body is different & nuanced. These suggestions are not meant to replace the guidance of an experienced healer or care-provider. I suggest perusing these options & persuing more information & access to whichever remedies feel most appropriate or appealing to you.

In addition to seeking counsel from a professional care-provider or trusted healer in your community, check in with your body for decision making! It is wiser than any book, google search, or doctor.

Main objectives for balancing the body:

- Manage Pain from Cramping

- Control Bleeding

- Build Blood

- Balance Hormone levels: both stress & sex

Acupuncture & Asian Bodywork

Acupuncture & Asian bodywork of various kinds rely on ancient & intelligent energy maps of the body. They are often based on assessing & assisting the flow of qi (life force) as well as elemental energies such as fire, earth, water, wind, & metal within the body. Acupuncture is one of my absolute favorite healing modalities as I have seen dramatic, powerful & tangible results from it both personally & professionally. The following are helpful in supporting every one of the main objectives for balancing the body listed above:

Acupuncture

A Chinese practice of stimulating flow of qi with needles placed gently (& generally shallowly & painlessly) in specific points.

Moxibustion

A Chinese practice of burning compressed bundles of the herb mugwort on or over specific points to stimulate qi flow & heat.

Acupressure

A Chinese & Japanese practice of stimulating flow of qi with massage & applied pressure to energy meridians in the body. Various forms include but are not limited to Amma, Shiatsu, Watsu, Tui Na.

Thai Bodywork

Very interactive stretching & pressure incorporating various traditions including yoga (recommend waiting a few weeks postpartum).

Herbs

There is a common misconception that herbs are always gentle. In fact, many of them are incredibly powerful & will create dramatic effects. Herbs can be taken in many forms, including but not limited to tinctures made from alcohol or glycerin, tea infusions, vinegar tonics, or capsules. Herbal baths infused with strong tea are a delightful way to immerse yourself in plant medicine's healing power.

Rosemary Gladstar, Aviva Romm, Susun Weed & Tori Hudson are some favorite sources for excellent herbal information for reproductive health. Ideally, consult an experienced herbalist in-person before beginning any herbal regimen.

Plant medicine demands thoughtful & respectful use. If you are interested in going deeper with plant medicine you may wish to pursue meditation or study delving into the clinical actions as well as sentient & spiritual properties of plants. One can benefit from creating a personal, intimate relationships with plants local to their area.

Pain Relievers

For cramps or inflammation.

Cramp Bark (Viburnum opulus)
Relaxes smooth muscle tissue, of which the uterus is made.

Jamaican Dogwood (Piscidia piscipula)
Anti-inflammatory, anti-spasmodic.

Silk Tassel (Garrya alliptica)
Anti-spasmodic (cramps are spasmodic!) & uterine stimulant.

Ginger & Cayenne
Along with other spicy/heating foods & herbs will improve circulation & thus decrease cramping.

Yellow Pond Lily (Nuphar lutea)
Pain reliever, pelvic tonic, & slows bleeding.

Ladies Mantle (Alchemilla millefolium)
Belongs in almost ALL the herbal categories listed in this book: astringent, tonic, reduces chance of hemorrhage.

Pulsatilla (Anemone pulsatilla)
Anti-spasmodic, pain reliever. Low dose botanical.

Black Cohosh (Cimicifuga/Actaea racemosa)
Pain reliever, antispasmodic; especially for pain in the lower back. This plant medicine is also a powerful psycho-spiritual healer of "underworld" experiences & is supportive of confronting darkness. Low dose botanical.

Wild Yam (Dioscorea villosa)
Anti-spasmodic especially associated with any stomach cramping, pain.

Pelvic Tonics

Tonify uterus & help it return to its normal state.

Raspberry (Rubus spp.)
Gentle tonic that nourishes the uterine muscles & lining, also high in minerals.

Yarrow (Achillea millefolium)
Slows bleeding, tonifies injured tissue.

Black Cohosh (Cimicifuga/Actaea racemosa)
Relaxes uterus, allows for the expulsion of the contents. Low dose botanical.

Blood Builders

High in minerals & nutrients.

Nettle (Urtica dioica)
High in iron & magnesium, also acts as a uterine tonic.

Yellow Dock (Rumex crispus)
Helps absorb iron, high in vitamin A, & potassium.

Yarrow (Achillea millefolium)
Rich in many minerals (also good for emotional boundary keeping & blood stasis).

Red Clover (Trifolium pratense)
High in many valuable nutrients including calcium, chromium, magnesium, niacin, phosphorus, potassium, thiamine, & vitamin C.

Red Clover (Trifolium pratense)
High in calcium.

Rehmannia glutinosa
Systemic regulating action on the blood mediated by building the liver.

Blood Stasis/Controlling Bleeding

Only use in cases of excessive blood loss.

Cinnamon Erigeron Tincture
Helps to slow bleeding, uterine tonic.

Yarrow (Achillea millefolium)
Stops bleeding, helps to heal wounds.

Crane's Bill (Geranium spp.)
Both a blood styptic & tonic, high in nutrients.

Yunnan Baiyao
A Chinese herb for use only in extreme cases of excessive bleeding or hemorrhage. Also a pain reliever, & said to help heal broken hearts/recover from trauma emotionally.

Shepard's Purse (Capsella bursa-pastoris)

Used in traditional midwifery & folk medicine to slow hemorrhage.

Adrenal Support

Herbs that support the function of the adrenal glands, which produce & regulate stress hormones, as well as relaxing herbs that help stress management & overall nervous system help. These are often referred to as "adaptogens."

The first three herbs are stimulating adaptogens & can be overly stimulating when consumed with caffeine.

Ashwagandha (Withania somnifera)

Nourishing adaptogen, helps build iron, & helps promote healthy hormonal cycles & balance.

Holy Basil (Ocimum sanctum)

A wonderful nourishing adaptogen with a vast history of use in India & Ayurvedic medicine. Sometimes called "Tulsi" which translates as "the incomparable one."

Eleuthero (Elutherococcus senticosus)

Also known as Siberian Ginseng. Powerful, complex, & safe adaptogen Chinese herbalists called "The King of the Adaptogens."

Rhodiola (Rhodiola rosea)

Adrenal tonic, improves hormone balance, & helps to heal injured tissue.

Ginseng (Panax ginseng)

Improves immunity, adrenal function, & energy.

Milky Oats (Avena sativa)

Nourishing tonic for adrenals, also high in minerals.

Rose (Rosa spp.)

Said to be "the highest vibration" flower, soothing, anti-depressant, helpful to the heart & emotional healing.

Catnip (Nepeta cataria)

Anti-anxiety, nervine.

Wood Betony (Stachys officinalis)

Anti-anxiety, nervine.

Lemon Balm (Melissa officinalis)

Anti-depressant.

St. John's Wort (Hypericum perforatum)

Calming nervine, anti-depressant; helpful to liver pathways that help with hormone regulation.

Motherwort (Leonurus cardiaca)

Bitter nervine, helps with anxiety & all aspects of emotional & energetic "mothering" — an energy we need to turn inward to nurture ourselves after abortion.

Immune Support

Herbs to help avoid & prevent infection.

Yerba Mansa (Anemopsis californica)

Anti-infectious, tonic.

Echinacea (Echinacea purpurea)

Anti-infectious, anti-inflammatory.

Oregon Grape (Mahonia aquifolium)

Anti-bacterial, antiviral, & tonic for mucous membranes.

Hormone Helpers

Herbs that help balance hormones.

Chaste Tree (Vitex agnus-castus)
   Helps stabilize progesterone.

Red Clover (Trifolium pratense)
   Excellent source of phytoestrogens.

Rhodiola (Rhodiola rosea)
   Adrenal tonic, improves hormone balance, & helps to heal injured tissue (Rhodiola can be too stimulating for some people, it is also a strong adaptogen).

Ashwagandha (Withania somnifera)
   Supports endocrine (hormone regulator) function, specifically supportive of thyroid function & helps lowers cortisol production. In India & Ayervedic medicine, Ashwagandha is known as the "strength of the stallion."

Heat

For pain relief, improved circulation & general coziness, place one of the following on your lower belly or back if that's where you're cramping. Cramping occurs due to ligaments connected to the uterus, as well as uterine contractions.

- Hot water bottle

- Rice/Buckwheat pillow warmed in the microwave

- Electric heating pad

- Warm Stones

Additional heat-based soothing measures may include:

- Immersion in a hot shower or bath

- Sauna

Vaginal Steams

Wait until you have had at least one full day without any bleeding or spotting to do a vaginal steam. If you do not wait until bleeding has ceased, you may prolong it.

Vaginal steaming is a very simple process that involves water, herbs, a blanket, a chair & about an hour of time. It is an ancient tradition practiced by Mayan & Asian cultures that both physically & energetically nourishes & cleanses the pelvic bowl. The essential oils from herbs vaporize into the steam & can positively affect the tissues of not only your vulva & vagina, but cervix & womb as well.

Any combination or individual use of the following herbs is appropriate:

- Oregano

- Basil

- Marigold

- Rosemary

- Burdock leaves

- Motherwort

- Chamomile

- Yarrow

- Plantain

- Lavender

- Thyme

Instructions for Vaginal Steaming:

- Simmer a handful of your chosen herbs for about ten minutes in a covered pot with 2 quarts of water on the stove/ over a fire, making a strong tea.

- Remove from heat & leave the lid on to catch the essential oils until you are ready to sit over the steam.

- Place the pot underneath a chair with slots or a mesh bottom that steam can penetrate. You may also clean your toilette & place tea in a bowl that fits snugly rested on the toilette bowl's edges, underneath the seat (usually used to make a "sitz bath"). You may also put tea in a container inside a bucket you sit on. Get creative!

- Take a seat (naked from the waist down) & wrap a blanket or large towel over your lap & around the chair/bucket/toilette seat to trap in all the steam.

- Relax & enjoy your healing vaginal steam anywhere from 20 minutes to an hour. This is great time to practice meditation techniques as well, or just enjoy a book or movie.

Nutrition

Nutritional healing is powerful healing. Getting your vitamins & minerals directly from organic & whole foods is optimal for absorption & integration! Take care to eat cooked & "warming" foods immediately after miscarriage & ideally for the next 40 days. Bone broths, ginger teas, & hot spiced drinking chocolate are all traditional things to feed people postpartum in various cultures, & are equally helpful post-miscarriage. The idea of keeping the body & especially womb space warm throughout the immediate postpartum period is nearly universal among many cultures around the world throughout history. Dressing warmly & consuming warming foods can help restore heat & energy to the body that was lost with the end of the pregnancy.

Iron & Vitamin C

- Dark leafies (especially when eaten or prepared with vinegar)

- Red fruits & veggies such as tomatoes, beets, berries

- Orange veggies like carrots, yams

- Red meat

- Tahini & sesame seeds are incredibly high in iron

- Seeds of all kinds are excellent nourishment, especially when sprouted

- Cooking in cast iron skillets adds significant nutritional value to the food

Zinc

For immune function & preventing infection.

- Shellfish & seafood, particularly oysters

- Cashews

- Chickpeas

Protein

For rebuilding tissue & sustainable energy.

- Meats (chicken, turkey, beef, pork)

- Fish, Seafood

- Tofu

- Lentils, cooked beans

- Quinoa

- Eggs

- Nuts & seeds

Supplements to Consider

Floradix
Iron & B vitamin complexes.

Magnesium
For cramping. Helps with muscle relaxation & healing. 2000 mg every few hours to digestive tolerance (discontinue use if you get diarrhea).

Calcium
Best taken in combination with magnesium.

Vitamin E

For wound healing & tissue repair, especially if the miscarriage was assisted with instruments inside the womb.

Bone Broths

Can be bought prepared or made at home. For making at home, use bones leftover from a meal or bought from a butcher (chicken, beef, turkey, whatever), add cold water & apple cider vinegar for bones to soak for 30 min. Then add vegetables to stock, bring to a boil, & reduce to simmer for 24–48 hours.

- Excellent source of minerals: calcium, phosphorus, magnesium & more.

- Rich in amino acids glycine & proline that assist in muscle & tissue repair, immune & nervous system function.

- Chondroitin sulphates & glucosamine found in bone broth reduce inflammation.

Movement

Dance

Any & all kinds. Belly dance is especially healing as it brings awareness, flow, & vital life energy into the pelvic bowl.

Qi Gong

Literally means "Life Energy Cultivation." It is a practice of aligning breath, movement & awareness for exercise, healing, & meditation.

Yoga

Restorative poses only for first 6 weeks. Look for a Yin or restorative style yoga classes or videos for instruction. Do gentle flowing yoga with rhythmic breathing & movements, nothing straining. It's recommended to wait 8–10 weeks postpartum for an active practice.

Moving in Nature

Walking, gentle hiking, gardening, wild crafting plant medicine, picnicking, etc.

Music

The benefits of music can be felt instantly. Rhythm & harmony literally heal & transform us through vibration. Music has been used by the healers & shamans of traditional cultures to cure illness & call in one's spirit home when it has been "lost" throughout history. The science of music therapy is an expanding & exciting field. A simple internet search can reveal numerous studies that complement the ancient wisdom of sound & song healing.

Music Has Been Found to Improve:

- Cardiovascular health

- Adrenal function

- Pain management

- Post-operative recovery

- Gastrointestinal health

- Metabolic health

- Vital energy

- Exercise recovery time

- Decrease stress hormones

- Decrease inflammation

Making music yourself can be wonderfully cathartic & healing, but at this time also consider just relaxing & receiving. Live music is best, but recordings will work too. Consider finding local healers who work with singing bowls, tuning forks, or other specific forms of music therapy if you'd like to explore therapeutic forms of music & vibration in greater depth.

Vocalizing & Toning

Vocalization & toning brings direct vibration through the body, tapping into your ability to heal yourself. Because these vibrations touch each of our cells, they may dredge up "hidden" feelings & emotions you may have not intellectually felt yet. This is normal! Be gentle & slow with yourself.

- Release through moaning, toning, singing, & talking.

- Deep singing & moaning produce vibrations in the body that affect all tissues, including the uterine muscles, therefore moaning & toning can physically relieve the uterine muscle cramping.

- "Sphincter Law" as described by Ina May Gaskin, also known as the hypoglossal pelvic nerve connection, explains the phenomena that when the throat & jaw are relaxed & open, the sphincter muscles down below are relaxed & open as well. Therefore, opening & relaxing your jaw, throat, & mouth can help release tension & trauma in the sphincter muscles of the pelvis, cervix, vagina & anus. Consider this in coping with moments of acute pain or cramping & for a regular healing practice if you have experienced trauma or tend to hold tension in your pelvis.

- To achieve greatest therapeutic effect from moaning & toning, lie down with a hand on your lower abdomen. Take a deep breath in, & release it with a deep low tone. Experiment with tones & the release of your breath. Eventually you will find one that creates the strongest vibration in your womb. You should be able to feel it with your hand through your belly. Stick with the tone that creates the highest vibration, taking deep breaths in between. Enjoy deeply & often!

- Take care to keep your jaw relaxed & mouth open (employing benefits of Sphincter Law).

Orgasm!

The healing power of orgasm & orgasmic energy cannot be over-stated! It is so good for you! Combining orgasm with elements of the toning/moaning practice described above can be very powerfully healing. Most clinical approaches suggest waiting a minimum of 1–2 weeks postpartum for penetration of anything into the vagina or until you have stopped bleeding completely as this introduces foreign bacteria into the vagina & potentially the womb, increasing risk of infection. Take your sweet time if you need longer than this. Some people find powerful heal-ing through sexual engagement earlier than this recommended timeline as well. Remember: delicious orgasms can be achieved by many without penetration as well!

Remember that the body can ovulate as soon as 1–2 weeks post-miscarriage. If your orgasmic practice also involves inter-acting with sperm, consider intentionality around potential conception. If a repeat pregnancy is undesired at this time, use contraception. While conceiving again right away may be attrac-tive to you, consider whether your body has had enough time to physically & emotionally heal to make a new nest for another pregnancy.

The physiologically healing benefits of orgasm include but are not limited to:

- Increases pelvic blood flow, lymph movement & circulation which eases cramps & helps tissue health.

- Releases the hormones dopamine, oxytocin, serotonin & endorphins from the brain, improving mood & reducing pain.

- Energizes your hypothalamus, which regulates appetite, body temperature, emotions, & the pituitary gland, which in turn regulates the release of reproductive hormones & helps reestablish a healthy cycle & fertility.

- Increases DHEA levels in the body. DHEA is a hormone precursor to estrogen & testosterone that improves brain function, balances the immune system, maintains & repairs tissues, & promotes healthy skin.

- Boosts infection-fighting cells up to 20%!

Aromatherapy & Essential Oils

Essential oils are amazingly powerful healing allies. Our sense of smell has been scientifically proven to provoke some of the most emotional reactions of any of our physical senses. I am quite wary of most internal uses of essential oils, & do not recommend it here for that reason. Some ways to use essential oils or aromatherapy healing include:

- Inhalation—Place a few drops in a pot of hot water or in your humidifier.

- In the bath—Add several drops to bathwater.

- Place a few drops on a hot compress (washcloth).

- Dilute in a carrier oil such as almond, coconut, or olive & use for massage.

- Diffuse into a room by heating in a special stand or gadget, or by simply simmering a few drops in a small open pot of water.

Some scents I recommend for this time include (but are not limited to):

Rose
  Anti-depressant, septic, viral, anti-inflammatory, anti-hemorrhage, uterine tonic, hormone balancer (especially great blended with geranium or lavender).

Geranium
  Uterine relaxant, anti-microbial, & regulator of uterine bleeding.

Lavender

Antiseptic, analgesic, anticonvulsant, anti-depressant, anti-rheumatic, antispasmodic, anti-inflammatory, antiviral, bactericide, carminative, cholagogue, cicatrisant, cordial, decongestant, deodorant, diuretic, emmenagogue, nervine, sedative.

Veriditas Botanicals Cramp Blend

Highly recommended effective blend for placing directly on abdomen for cramp relief (many other brands have similar blends, I just love this one).

Cinnamon

To restore & bring heat to the body & senses.

Helichrysum (sometimes called Everlasting)

Blood mover & anti-bruising (moving out dead cells & in healing white blood cells).

Belly Binding

Belly binding has been used in many different traditional cultures throughout history, including West Africa, South America, & Asia to support people through pregnancy & postpartum. Many of these cultures have intricate or special ways of wrapping material to support bellies both healing & strengthening.

There's no need to use special technique or expensive cloth to enjoy the benefits of extra heat & support from wrapping your belly in cloth after pregnancy loss. A snuggly wrapped shawl or scarf can be wonderfully supportive & comforting to the womb space & muscles supporting & surrounding it. Cross culturally, bringing extra heat to the womb is an important protocol for easing discomfort during menstruation, pregnancy, & postpartum. Wrapping yourself after pregnancy termination is a simple way to care for yourself & remind yourself that you are healing. 40 days is a common period of time to wrap postpartum, but continue the practice as long as it feels good to you.

Womb & Pelvic Health

While there are many varieties of healing touch that may be benficial, from snuggling to Swedish Massage to Shiatsu, I wanted to include mention of these two special (& lesser known) womb-centric modalities. A minimum of six weeks postpartum is recommended before receiving a treatment.

Holistic Internal Pelvic Massage

Addresses physical & energetic imbalances that block or limit a person's pelvic energy, creative aspirations, or core vitality, including intervaginal massage, myofascial release, trigger point work, & visualization tools for regaining balance.

Arvigo Technique of Mayan Abdominal Massage

An external massage working to restore the body to its natural balance by correcting the position of organs that have shifted & restrict the flow of blood, lymph, nerve, & energy, focused on the womb & abdominal area. Usually includes instruction in self-massage for continued self-care.

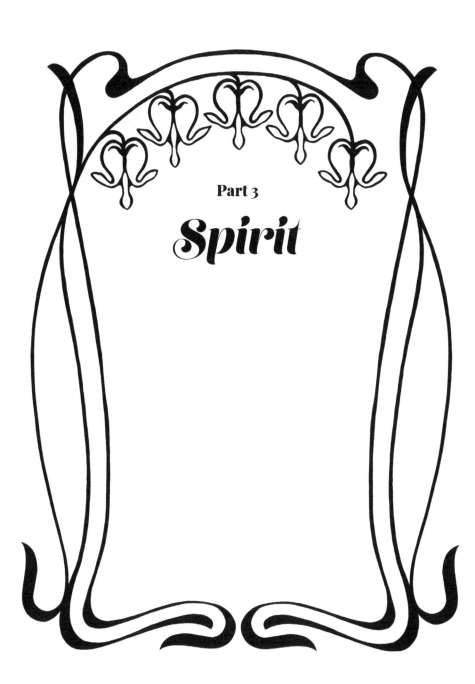

Part 3

Spirit

"Birth & death are not two different states, but they are different aspects of the same state."

Ghandi

Amidst the likelihood of pain & grief, miscarriage presents an opportunity for profound transformation & reverence for life. The womb is a spirit door. In regaining balance from pregnancy loss we have the opportunity to intentionally examine, define, & manifest our connection with divine creative energy implicit in our bodies.

Meditation

Meditation can foster feelings of expansiveness, calm, & connectivity. It can be practiced solo or in community. Any action can be an act of meditation if it is done with spiritual presence & intention. There are many options & types of structured meditation including but not limited to:

Breathing
Various patterns & exercises with our breath affect our state of mind & emotions.

Visualization
Focusing on particular calming, meaningful, or beautiful images in our mind's eye.

Mindfulness/Zazen/Vispassana
Seated simplistic Buddhist traditions.

Kundalini
Cultivating & connecting to a feminine life force energy stream in our body, assisting its flow from the base of our spine through the head.

Qi Gong
Literally means "Life Energy Cultivation", a Chinese practice of aligning breath, movement & awareness for exercise, healing, & meditation.

Walking Meditation & Labyrinths

Engaging in soft, steady walking whilst working to clear the mind to a meditative state, often done in a labyrinth or other specific pattern in a designated space.

Hypnosis

Trance states for transforming habits & elements of our subconscious, usually induced by an experienced practitioner, though can be explored in the self alone.

Mantras or Affirmations

Focusing on & repeating a healing statement.

Artistic Expression

Any kind of visual art, writing, dance, or craft can serve this purpose. All of life is art if you view it as such!

Express yourself!
Create!

If you're making physical objects or drawings, you can choose to keep them, or consider enjoying the catharsis of destroying them with or without a ritual surrounding the act. Burning & burying are some options for cathartic destruction.

A Liminal Letter

An excellent artistic exercise I recommend is writing a letter with your non-dominant hand to yourself from a choice of: ·

· Your "higher self."

· The spirit you have just released from your womb.

· Your physical womb personified.

Imagine what these entities would say to you if they could speak. What would they want you to know? This process can help connect you with & express energies from a more emotional & spiritual perspective that is less linear or rational.

Ritual

Ritual is something that creates a separation from daily life, makes sacred space, & connects with & honors Spirit. It is most important that ritual has personal meaning. It does not have to follow a set formula from any suggestion, faith, prescribed ceremony, or other source. Below are simply some suggestions, but as always, you know best. Consult your intuition.

To Create a Custom Ritual

1. Plan & Clarify Intention

- Who: Humans to be present, &/or deity/spirits to be invoked.

- What: Objects, elements, colors, symbols.

- Where: What space & location?

- Why: Create a clear statement of intention.

2. Create Sacred Space & Open the Ritual

- Make an alter space with physical items or symbols of importance to you.

- Burn incense &/or clearing plants (ex: cedar, Palo Santo, sage).

- Call the directions.

- Casting a circle (salt, cornmeal, or visualization are some tools for this).

- State your intention.

- Light candles.

3. Grounding—use a meditation or physical action to connect with the earth.

- Become fully present in your body.

4. Action

- Create.

- Burn, bury, smash symbolic objects or artwork.

- Song, dance, chanting.

- Meditation.

5. Closing of the Ritual/Opening of Circle

- Release & thank any energies invoked (including self).

- Cleanse self & or circle with same or different action as opening.

Traditional Ceremonies

The following are just a few ceremonies that I am familiar with, there are many more to seek & find. It is my hope that some of these concepts or practices will inspire a felt experience of resonance, reverence, or self awareness for you. As you explore the lineages & traditions of bloodlines that do not belong to you, please do so with respect for the nuanced difference between appropriation & appreciation.

Even if you are not a regular member of these communities or "believer" of the faith, the integrity & richness of these ancient traditions can support you in your time of need. You may want to seek out an experienced guide from one of these heritages or faiths, or research the options & adapt them creatively to your individual needs.

Burial/Funeral

Across many cultures & practices both ancient & modern, many honor their dead with burial. Some may find comfort in the ritual of a burial after a pregnancy loss, either of blood & tissue or of a symbolic offering like an egg, seed, special flower, or other artifact related to the pregnancy. Some cemeteries have designated space for pregnancy loss, others may consider their own land or another special garden or space.

Ceremony to Release Spirit Life

A tradition from the Taino Clan, native to the Caribbean islands that includes ritual ceremonial bath, songs to the Grandmothers & Guardian Spirit, & a dreaming of the spirit life back into the Great Womb where all spirits go at the end of life.

Closing of the Bones Ceremony

A traditional Mexican/Mayan ceremony involving massage, ritual herb bath, & being wrapped tightly in rebozos, or shawls. It is meant to create a feeling of multi-dimensional closure & integrity after transition &/or loss.

Mizuko Kuyo Ceremony

Traditional Japanese Zen Buddhist practice honoring a returning of babies lost in pregnancy & early years of life back to the water of the river that divides realms of life & death/rebirth. Involving special words, blessings, & red gifts to statues of Jizo, the bodhisattva that protects & cares for lost babies in their transition.

Mikvah

A traditional Jewish bathing ritual for renewal, rebirth, cleansing & transformation.

Offerings of Red Eggs

Predating Christianity & Easter Traditions, red-dyed eggs were once offered in cemeteries in Eastern Europe, particularly Slavic traditions, to commemorate miscarriages & stillbirths.

Mother Roasting

An anthropological term describing a collection of postpartum practices in China & Southeast Asia (each distinct within cultural regions) involving warm baths, belly binding, confinement to the home, special warming diets, etc. for a designated amount of time after a birth. Could be equally applicable after a loss.

Resources

This list is constantly evolving. For the most up-to-date resource list, please see my website www.samanthazipporah.com

Books

Miscarriage

- Heustis, Jane, Marcia Meyers Jenkins, and Alan D. Wolfelt. *Companioning at a Time of Perinatal Loss: A Guide for Nurses, Physicians, Social Workers, Chaplains and Other Bedside Caregivers.* Companion Press, 2004.

- Ilse, Sherokee. *Empty Arms: Coping with Miscarriage, Stillbirth and Infant Death.* Edited by Arlene Applebaum. Wintergreen Press, 2013.

- Keating, Catherine Noblitt. *There Was Supposed To Be A Baby: A Guide to Healing After Pregnancy Loss.* Seattle, WA: Hummingbird Press, 2012.

- Kluger-Bell, Kim. *Unspeakable Losses: Understanding the Experience of Pregnancy Loss, Miscarriage, and Abortion.* 2000.

- Kohn, Ingrid, and Perry-Lynn Moffitt. *Pregnancy Loss: A Silent Sorrow: Guidance and Support for You and Your Family.* Place of Publication Not Identified: Headway, 1994.

- LeMoine, Monica Murphy. *Knocked Up, Knocked Down: Postcards of Miscarriage & Other Misadventures from the Brink of Parenthood.* Catalyst Book Press, 2010.

- Trautman, Kerry. *Mourning Sickness: Stories and Poems about Miscarriage, Stillbirth, and Infant Loss.* Edited by Missy Martin and Jesse Loren. Omni Arts, LLC, 2008.

- Moulder, Christine. *Miscarriage Women's Experiences and Needs.* London: Routledge, 2001.

- Panuthos, Claudia, and Catherine Romeo. *Ended Beginnings: Healing Childbearing Losses*. New York: Warner Books, 1986.

- *To Linger on Hot Coals: Collected Poetic Works from Grieving Women Writers*. Place of Publication Not Identified: Strategic Book Publishing, 2014.

Ritual & Ceremony

- Bays, Jan Chozen. Jizo Bodhisattva: *Guardian of Children, Travelers, & Other Voyagers*. Shambala, 2003.

- Beck, Renee, and Sydney Barbara Metrick. *The Art of Ritual: Creating and Performing Ceremonies for Growth and Change*. Berkeley, CA: Apocryphile Press, 2009.

- Lamb, Jane Marie. *Bittersweet—Hellogoodbye*. Belleville, IL: Charis Communications, 1988.

- Maia, Deborah, and Sudie Rakusin. *Self-ritual for Invoking Release of Spirit Life in the Womb: A Personal Treatise on Ritual Herbal Abortion*. Great Barrington, MA: Mother Spirit, 1989.

- Makichen, Walter. *Spirit Babies*. Random House USA, 2005.

- Peterson, Aileen. *Rituals & Meditations for Pregnancy Release*. 13 Moons of Matrescence.

- Vesta, Lara. *The Moon Divas Guidebook: Spirited Self-Care for Women in Transition*. Portland, OR: Inkwater Press, 2012.

Holistic Health

- Gage, Suzann, Sylvia Morales, and Katharina Allers. *A New View of a Womans Body: A Fully Illustrated Guide*. Los Angeles: Feminist Health Press, 1995.

- Northrup, Christiane. *Womens Bodies Womens Wisdom: Creating Physical and Emotional Health and Healing*. New York: Bantam Books, 2002.

- The Boston Women's Health Book Collective. *Our Bodies Ourselves*. Touchstone Books: 1998.

- Clark, Demetria. *Aromatherapy and Herbal Remedies for Pregnancy, Birth, & Breastfeeding*. Summertown, TN: Book Publishing Company, 2015.

- David, Marc. *Nourishing Wisdom: A New Understanding of Eating*. New York: Bell Tower, 1991.

- Fallon, Sally, Mary G. Enig, Kim Murray, and Marion Dearth. *Nourishing Traditions: The Cookbook That Challenges Politically Correct Nutrition and the Diet Dictocrats*. Washington, DC: NewTrends Publishing, 2005.

- Moskowitz, Richard. *Homeopathic Remedies for Pregnancy & Childbirth*. 1993.

- Romm, Aviva Jill. *The Natural Pregnancy Book: Your Complete Guide to a Safe, Organic Pregnancy and Childbirth with Herbs, Nutrition, and Other Holistic Choices*. Berkeley: Ten Speed Press, 2014.

Websites

Community & Stories

unspokengrief.com
tinyfootprintsonmyheart.wordpress.com
nationalshare.org
fullspectrumdoulacircle.com

Selected Articles

- "How to Help a Friend Deal With Miscarriage" Jezebel.com article.

- "Mothering Yourself Through A Miscarriage" SQUAT Birth Journal article.

- "Hope Is Born With Every Loss" SQUAT Birth Journal article.

- "The Energetic Placenta: Healing From Abortion & Miscarriage" healingwithouteffort.com article.

- "People Have Misconceptions About Miscarriage, & That Can Hurt" npr.org article.

- "A Transgender Patient in the ER: 12 Hours" (on miscarriage, hospital treatment, & trans* bodies) milkjunkies.com article.

Ritual for Pregnancy Loss & Termination
spiritbabies.org

Financial Assistance for Funeral Arrangements
thetearsfoundation.org

All Options & Pregnancy Experiences Hotline
Backline 1-888-493-0092
yourbackline.org

About the Author

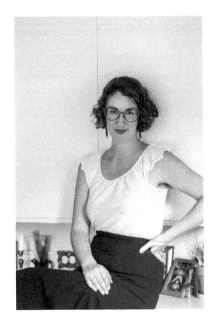

Samantha Zipporah is a fertility & sexuality educator, activist, & advocate. She teaches body literacy & walks a path of service to womb sovereignty. She believes the mind, body, & spirit connection deserve reverence & respect. Friends have joked that her business tagline should be, "If anything's going in or out of a cervix, call Sam."

A former birth doula whose roots of study can be found in traditional midwifery "womb to tomb" style care, Sam provides counsel for a diverse array of fertility, sexuality, & pregnancy experiences. Her approach is grounded in a solid understanding of biochemistry & biology, & nourished by playfulness, sass, & reverent spirituality.

To learn more about Sam & her work please visit her at www.samanthazipporah.com & follow her on social media.

Appendix A

Holistic Healing
Practitioners & Professionals

While almost all of the suggestions in this booklette can be self-administered, in some cases people may seek the care of a community healer or holistic healing professional. The following is a basic list of various holistic healers & professionals who may be of assistance after a miscarriage to look for in your community.

Possible professional credentials are listed to help narrow your search but are not meant to limit your search. There are many inspiring community healers without professional credentials.

Acupuncturist (L.Ac/R.Ac)
A practitioner specializing in acupuncture, or inserting small needles along energy meridians in keeping with Chinese medicinal ideology.

Aromatherapist
A practitioner specializing in essential oils & other methods of aromatherapy.

Clinical Thai Bodywork Practitioner (CTBP)
A massage therapist specializing in the unique forms of Thai bodywork.

Counsellor/Therapist (especially ones who may work with hypnosis, somatic therapy, art therapy)
Could range from talk therapy to art or movement based therapy, but counsellors/therapist are usually trained in psychology & helping an individual heal through working on internal thoughts & reframing.

Dance Instructor (all kinds!)
Any kind of dance/instructor that appeals to you.

Doula/Full Spectrum Doula
Doulas usually attend clients through pregnancy, birth & postpartum offering informational & physical (non-medical) support & guidance. "Full spectrum" doulas particularly serve clients of all pregnancy outcomes, including pregnancy loss.

Flower Essence & Vibrational Healing Practitioner
Those who specialize in assessing for most appropriate flower essence for healing.

Herbalist
A practitioner specializing in plant-based medicinal preparations for healing. Herbalism is largely unregulated in most of North America.

Homeopath (C.Hom)
A practitioner specializing in the quantum medicine of homeopathy .

Massage Therapist (including Shiatsu, Deep Tissue, Mayan Abdominal Massage, Holistic Internal Pelvic Massage, etc.)
Infinite varieties of healing touch.

Meditation Teacher/Mentor/Guide (of many kinds)
There are infinite branches, schools, & ways to practice mind-calming meditation, with many different kinds of practitioners.

Midwife (CPM, LM, RM, CNM, TM)
Traditional primary care providers for pregnancy, birth, postpartum, & early newborn care. Many midwives are skilled at managing pregnancy loss.

Musician
Performers, instructors, & musical healers.

Naturopathic Doctor (ND)
Specializing in comprehensive holistic health care with training in many of these modalities, many can also prescribe certain pharmaceutical medications.

Nutritionist (many different types, credentials)
Nutritionists & dieticians may give well-rounded advice on diets for certain times of life or for general wellness.

QiGong Instructor
Often also Chinese Medical Doctors, Reiki Practitioners, or other energy healing modality practitioners.

Reiki Master
Using light touch & energetic healing, often on a massage table.

Sexologist
Often a therapist or counselor, but not always, specializing in sex therapy & sexuality.

Shaman
Traditional spiritual support & guide in many cultures.

Spiritual Healer
Encompassing a wide variety of possible spiritual healing techniques.

Traditional Chinese Medicine (TCM) Practitioner/Chinese Medical Doctor (R.TCM.P/L.TCM.P)
Specializing in herbal preparations, other healing substances, & often acupuncture & acupressure.

Yoga Instructor
Many different styles of yoga & yoga teachers

Appendix B

Glossary of Terms

Absorption
The process of absorbing or being absorbed into the body.

Acupuncture
A Chinese tradition of healing based on redirecting qi energy flow along meridians in the body using needles inserted into the skin at specific points.

Acupressure
A multi-origin tradition of healing based on redirecting energy in the body by pressing on certain pressure points with the thumb or fingers.

Adaptogen
A plant extract able to increase the body's ability to resist the damaging effects of stress & restore normal physiological functioning.

Adrenal
Adrenal glands located near the kidneys help regulate hormones, particularly stress hormones.

Affirmation
A positive assertion designed to aid in meditation & psychological healing.

Altar
A designated sacred space, often on a table, where offerings may be left for honoring.

Amma
Ancient Chinese acupressure bodywork.

Analgesic

Pain-reliever.

Aromatherapy

The use of specific scents, often through essential oils, to aid in healing & altering moods & brain states.

Astringent

Helps tighten body tissues.

Belly binding

Wrapping the abdomen to invoke a "closed" feeling postpartum/post-loss.

Bodhisattva

A sacred being, capable of attaining enlightenment, that forgoes entering nirvana in order to help others on the path to enlightenment (Mahayana Buddhism).

Cardiovascular

Relating to the heart, blood vessels, & circulatory system between them.

Carminative

Expels gas from the intestines so as to relieve pain from abdominal swelling or flatulence.

Cathartic

Relief from releasing strong emotions. In herbal medicine, an herb that accelerates defecation.

Cholagogue

Promotes an increased flow of bile.

Cicatrisant

Promoting wound healing.

Cordial

An invigorating or stimulating medicine.

Anti-convulsant
Works against seizures or other involuntary muscle contractions.

Decongestant
A agent that relieves excessive accumulation of mucous.

Deity
A holy, divine, or sacred being.

Diuretic
Increases urine output.

Dopamine
A neurotransmitter the helps regulate the brain's reward & pleasure centers.

Emmenagogue
Promotes menstruation.

Endorphins
A peptide in the brain that bonds primarily to opioids for pain relief.

Essential oils
Volatile oil extracts made through steam distillation, expression, & extraction.

Flower essences
Infusions of wildflowers in spring water & sunlight with grape alcohol or brandy preservative to enhance subtle emotional healing.

Gastrointestinal
Relating to the stomach, intestines, & digestive tract.

Glycerin
Non-alcoholic medicine-making preservative.

Hemorrhage
Excessive blood loss.

Holistic
Honoring & integrating the mind, body, & spirit.

Homeopathy
A system of medicine originating in Germany in which treatment is based on the administration of minute doses of a remedy that would in healthy persons produce symptoms similar to those of the disease, promoting the body to heal itself.

Humidifier
Mechanical device for producing steam/mist & humidity in a room.

Hypnosis
A trancelike state of altered consciousness induced by a practitioners whose suggestions are readily accepted by the subject.

Inflammation (anti-inflammatory)
Reduces redness, heat, swelling as a reaction to injury or infection.

Infusion
Steeping or soaking in water in order to extract certain constituents.

Invoke
To call forth, or make an earnest request for.

Kundalini
Yogic life force lying at the base of the spine.

Labyrinth
An elaborate structure with winding, patterned paths leading to a center & then returning to the start. Distinct from a maze, a labyrinth only has one path, however intricate, & one cannot get lost.

Ligaments
Tough muscle tissue in the body that holds organs in place or bones together.

Lymph
Pale bodily fluid containing white blood cells that maintains healthy tissues.

Mantra
A repeated phrase in prayer or meditation.

Meditation
A wide variety of practices usually focused on quiet clearing of daily thoughts.

Meridians
In Chinese medicine, paths through which life-energy flows.

Metabolic
Relating to the chemical changes in cells by which energy is provided for vital processes & activities.

Mindfulness
The practice of maintaining a heightened awareness of one's thoughts, emotions, & experiences on a moment-to-moment basis.

Miscarriage
The loss of a pregnancy before the developing embryo/fetus/baby has reached "viability" (ability to live autonomously outside the womb).

Moxibustion
In Chinese or Japanese medicine the use of mugwort herbal bundles to introduce heat to specific points or acupuncture needles.

Nervine
Soothes nervous excitement or stimulation.

Ovulate
The release of a mature ovum (egg) from the ovary into the fallopian tube in hopes of fertilization.

Progesterone
A hormone stimulating & promoting growth especially of the endometrium (uterine lining) before menstruation & in early pregnancy.

Prolactin
A hormone that induces lactation.

Anti-pyretic
Prevents or reduces fever.

Qi
In Chinese Medicine, "life force energy."

Qi Gong
Chinese healthcare practice involving postures, movement, breathing techniques, & focused intention.

Reiki
Focused, light touch/bodywork designed to redirect energy fields & flow & promote healing.

Anti-rheumatic
Helps relieve rheumatism/arthritis.

Sauna
Special heated room for sweating out toxins in the body.

Sedative
Calms, moderates, or tranquilizes nervousness & excitement.

Sentient
Conscious.

Antiseptic
Against bacterial infection.

Serotonin

Neurotransmitter responsible for transmitting impulses between nerve cells, regulating cyclical body processes, & contributing to feelings of happiness.

Shiatsu

Japanese acupressure involving pressure points, massage, & joint manipulation.

Singing bowl

An inverted bell shaped as a bowl conducting vibrational sound, especially in Buddhist practices.

Antispasmodic

Controls muscle spasms.

Stimulant

Increasing energy.

Styptic

Contract or bind, especially to stop bleeding.

Thai bodywork

Combines bodywork, massage, Ayurvedic principles & assisted yoga postures.

Tuning fork

A metal device with two long points that when struck produces a certain note/vibration.

Tonics

Promoting health muscular condition & retraction of organs/ solution of herbs & carrier water/oil/molasses/etc. to promote above body tone.

Toning

Using your voice to express specific sounds or tones that help you to release, balance, accept, or create.

Tui Na

Chinese healing practice using body manipulation based in Taoist & martial arts principles.

Vaginal steams

Bringing concentrated heat/steam infused with herbs to the vulva to promote healing & connection.

Vipassana

Ancient Indian technique of meditation.

Wat su

Aquatic bodywork used for deep relaxation & passive aquatic therapy.

Wildcrafting

Specific set of ethical principles applies to harvesting plants & herbs from the wild.

Yoga

An Indian/Hindu practice of experiencing inner peace by controlling the mind & body, often expressed through a series of bodily poses.

Zazen

Seated meditation in Japanese Zen Buddhism.

"I'm great at a deathbed. I've never given tranquilisers or psychiatric medicine. I've given love & fun & creativity & passion & hope, & these things ease suffering."

Patch Adams